Improving Students' Motivation to Study

A Photocopiable Resource for College and University Lecturers

Improving Students' Motivation to Study

A Photocopiable Resource for College and University Lecturers

Tim Duffy and Russell Rimmer

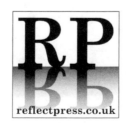

Reflect Press Ltd
www.reflectpress.co.uk

First published in 2008

ISBN: 978 1 906052 11 9

British Library Cataloguing in Publication Data
A catalogue record for this book is available from the British Library

Production project management by Deer Park Productions, Tavistock, Devon

Typeset by TW Typesetting, Plymouth, Devon

Cover design by Oxmed

Printed and bound by Ashford Colour Press, Gosport, Hants

Distributed by BEBC, Albion Close, Parkstone, Poole, Dorset BH12 3LL

Reflect Press Ltd
www.reflectpress.co.uk
Published by Reflect Press Ltd
11 Attwyll Avenue
Exeter
Devon, EX2 5HN
UK
01392 204400

Contents

Acknowledgements

The authors and publisher would like to thank Emeritus Professor Noel Entwistle for permission to use items from the *Approaches and Study Skills Inventory for Students* (ASSIST) and Professor Angus Duff for permission to use 20 items from the *Revised Approaches to Studying Inventory* (RASI) in the SAMI.

Author Biographies

Dr Tim Duffy

Tim Duffy is Director of Distance Learning within the School of Health, Nursing and Midwifery at the University of the West of Scotland. He is a qualified social worker and specialised in working with people with alcohol and drug-related problems. For six years he was National Training Officer with responsibility for training social work and health care personnel to develop strategies to motivate clients and patients to tackle alcohol- and drug-related problems. During this time he regularly delivered programmes focussing on motivational interviewing, problem solving and goal setting. He evaluated the effectiveness of this training and also the effectiveness of a minimal intervention for people with alcohol problems.

Since 1995 he has supported the development, delivery and evaluation of a range of undergraduate and post-graduate programmes. In this role he has supported students to focus and improve their approaches to study. His PhD study evaluated the impact of the SAMI in a UK Higher Education setting. This study borrowed and built on techniques used to motivate clients with alcohol and drug problems and applied them to students wishing to improve their approaches to study. The framework and effectiveness of this brief intervention is outlined in this book. Tim is currently researching student learning styles and approaches to study, student motivation, methods of supporting students online and student retention.

Professor Russell Rimmer

Russell Rimmer is Associate Dean and Head of Learning and Teaching in the School of Business, Enterprise and Management at Queen Margaret University. He has held positions in 'old' and 'new' universities in the UK and Australia and has taught on programmes in management, decision-making, economics, mathematics, science, applied statistics and research methods. Russell's research encompasses the economics of structural change with emphasis on the roles of education and training, the effectiveness of higher education initiatives and the career development of non-traditional entrants to universities. He is currently researching the relationships between student behaviour, decision-making, study effort and academic outcomes and how these prepare graduates for modern careers.

Improving Students' Motivation to Study

1. INTRODUCTION

The intention of this book is to provide a resource that can be used by students to improve their approaches to study in colleges and universities. This resource is known as the SAMI – Self Administered Motivational Instrument. Students can use the SAMI unaided by lecturers or tutors or they can be guided efficiently through it in terms of staff and class time. The SAMI has already been evaluated in the higher education sector and found to have positive effects on study habits and on academic performance.

The SAMI is a brief intervention that draws on motivational interviewing, learning-style theory and analytical decision-making. As far as the authors could discern, the SAMI is among the first brief instruments that draw on the principles of motivational interviewing to provide a means for college and university students to reflect on changing their approaches to study. Further, it is the first such intervention that is provided as a self-completing, self-help guide. The evidence is that people instigate successful change on their own or with relatively little assistance. In particular, many students can be assisted to change their study behaviour with the SAMI at little cost to the institutions in which they study. Students can complete the SAMI in around 30 minutes, which, for those with many demands on their time, is a considerable advantage. Moreover, by using the SAMI, students are unlikely to become stigmatised as they might if they were 'sent' to a specialist or remedial unit.

These advantages of the SAMI are of considerable value in modern post-school education. Across most of the Western world, governments are expanding opportunities for further and higher education, while funding to underpin expansion is limited. Further, there is ample evidence that post-school students are now more diverse in terms of observable characteristics, such as the number of years and quality of completed school education, and unobservable characteristics, such as their capacities to cope with the demands of study and other factors in their lives, such as work and families. The changing make-up of college and university intakes is discussed in the next section. In Section 3, the theory of the

SAMI is discussed and in Section 4 its design and layout are described. The practicalities of how to distribute, apply and use the SAMI are considered in Sections 5 and 6. Finally, in Section 7, concluding remarks are provided on the development and evaluation of the SAMI to date. Section 7 also includes an invitation to become involved in the ongoing development and research on approaches that use the SAMI framework.

2. THE EDUCATIONAL CONTEXT

2.1 Deepening and broadening the skill base

Over recent decades, governments have emphasised the economic role of post-secondary education in providing a highly skilled workforce. In many countries the political message has been received as confirmation of the view that a degree is required to get on in the world. Consequently, school leavers have increasingly taken up full-time higher education (HE). Others have taken routes that lead, via colleges of further education (FE), to articulation or advanced entry into degree programmes. These may be 'uninterrupted' routes in that a school leaver arrives at either FE or HE at the earliest opportunity after finishing secondary school and studies year on year until graduation.

Along with the economic imperative of skilling, governments have actively encouraged HE study among those who 'traditionally' did not participate.

'Non-traditional' entrants include:

- citizens who are older than 21 when they first consider HE;
- those who are of low socio-economic standing;
- citizens living in localities where few residents attend or have attended university;
- those who are disabled;
- citizens from racial or ethnic minorities.

The effect on the age of university entrants is striking in the UK. Over the years 1971 to 1973, less than four per cent of university entrants were older than 25; 25 years later, 25 per cent were over 25 (Woodley *et al.*, 1992; Richardson and Woodley, 2003).

2.2 Effort and academic outcomes

The drive to widen participation in post-school education has broadened the mix of student characteristics, such as age and socio-economic standing. Further, widening participation and the general acceptance of needing a degree to get on has wrought substantial variation and change in intrinsic characteristics. For example, evidence from Australia and the USA suggests that over the past three decades student effort has come to vary widely, while 'being well-off financially' has come to be a more important value among college students than 'developing a meaningful philosophy of life' (Astin, 1998; McInnes, 2001).

Study effort may vary more because many students now have few financial resources to support them. Thus, many students must 'work to live'. Of course, it is possible that other students choose to 'work to maintain lifestyle' (McInnes, 2001) – working to buy clothes, run cars, pay for entertainment and finance holiday travel. Whether to maintain life or lifestyle, study competes with work and other interests for time and effort (Callendar, 2005). Further, HE students in the UK and Australia choose how much study effort to apply in light of information on academic performance, which comes in the form of feedback on assignments and earlier tests or examinations (Houston, Knox and Rimmer, 2007; Donnelly, McCormack and Rimmer, 2007).

Students might decide, for example, that doing the assessable work in a second-semester module is pointless because the grades attained in the first-semester predecessor were poorer than expected. They would prefer to study those modules/units where they are certain they can attain passes and possibly also satisfy progression rules (QAA, 2004). Students who reduce study time in this way have the option of working or pursuing other activities in the time that they have freed up. However, students who take these decisions are left with modules they must pass at some future time. They may reason that these can be picked up by enrolling in more than a full-time load in a later semester or by extending the time they take to complete a degree (SQW, 2006).

The decision to reduce effort may not be as extreme as abandoning all assessments in one or more modules. Students can decide to attempt enough of the assessments in a module to ensure that a bare pass will be awarded. Alternatively, they might aim for sufficient marks to ensure they fulfil rules on satisfactory progress or to warrant a re-sit. Evidence gathered by one of the current authors indicates that mature part-time students who have family commitments might decide to aim for bare passes. This occurs also among traditional first-level entrants (Duffy, 2005).

At one Scottish university, which has widened participation beyond the benchmarks set by government, Houston and Rimmer (2005; 2007) have demonstrated that entrants who make less effort, in the form of attempting assessments in fewer modules, attain worse marks on average than do those who attempt assessments in more modules; and that worse marks are associated with reduced study effort in subsequent semesters. That is, students tend to 'disengage from' (McInnes, 2001; Houston et al., 2007) or not 'integrate into' (Tinto, 1975) post-school study. Across Australian universities McInnes (2001) acknowledged that this trend was also apparent. In the US, Kuh (1998; 2001) reported that students have developed a culture of entitlement; they appear to be getting better grades, while making less efforts than in the past; they have only occasional contact with lecturers and they spend about half of the time expected in preparing for classes.

2.3 Trading off study, work and life

2.3.1 Work and the financial costs of study

While there may be evidence that students have become more materialistic or strategic in their outlooks (McInnes, 2001; Donnelly *et al.*, 2007), this does not explain the reasoning underpinning the decisions they take or the contexts within which they reduce study effort. Further, it does not point lecturers, tutors and teachers towards how to engender greater engagement with study.

In many parts of the world, governments are asking full-time students and their families to share the expense of paying for higher education. For example, in England, Northern Ireland and Wales, governments have introduced tuition fees, while not necessarily ensuring that those with few economic resources are protected from the full impact this new obligation can have on them. For those who must 'work to live', tuition fees are likely to be a factor in decisions to work more (Brennan *et al.*, 2005). That is, it is understandable that pressure to work has increased and that modern students are more likely to work than traditional students did in the past.

2.3.2 Work experience, career development and career breaks

Undoubtedly, debt and work are major influences on the forms of engagement with post-school study forged by many students. However, there are others, each of relevance to particular groups of students and each of which can affect behaviour and study effort. Consider older students entering HE in their forties or fifties. When at school their experiences may have been less than satisfactory. This might be because of attitudes at the time to prolonged education for those from lesser socio-economic backgrounds. For older women, the attitudes to their initial schooling may have been very different from current attitudes to female learning. This may engender uncertainty about why they returned to education and may make the establishment of effective study patterns difficult. Moreover, Schuller and Bamford (2000, p. 13) record as impediments to women's further study 'explicit and implicit discouragement', such as initially supportive partners later taking different attitudes, 'negative peer pressure' and 'reactionary attitudes'.

The sorts of work experience that mature entrants bring to their studies can be of varying relevance. Women over 21 enrolling in business and management awards might not have experience to bring to their studies. For example, they may have worked as clerks or secretaries, sales assistants and waiters or bar staff. Male returners more frequently bring managerial experience to their studies (Houston and Rimmer, 2005). Women's experiences in business and management are likely to have been punctuated by breaks from work for family formation (ibid.). On the other hand, those enrolling at university as mature entrants in science, ICT and engineering disciplines are likely to have experience relevant to their studies (ibid.).

Overall, it is probable that the type of experience can influence study patterns and engagement. However, this can depend on the reasons for undertaking further or higher education. For example, many nurses in the UK who originally trained 'on the job' in hospitals, now enrol in HE to top up their initial qualifications to degree level. It may be that reasons to do with keeping up pay progression or not being overlooked for promotion, rather than intrinsic interest in learning and refining skills, are paramount. This may impact on study effort, in that 'doing just enough to pass' is thought to be sufficient. Similar considerations have been suggested as permeating the thinking of MBA students (Pfeffer and Fong, 2004; Reeves and Rimmer, 2008).

2.3.3 Family life

After the birth of children, mothers tend to be responsible for domestic concerns, even those who return to paid work (Rimmer and Rimmer, 1997). This is likely to persist when wives and mothers take up study. By contrast, older men returning to study may only need to fit their studies around the demands of employers.

Not only is there a gender dimension to engaging with study, there are interaction effects involving age (Houston et al., 2007). Younger women with little children may have frequent distractions from the study efforts they are prepared to make (Donnelly et al., 2007). Women in their forties or fifties may find that their children recognise the pressures involved in study and are supportive of them. Other women in their forties and fifties may be involved in the care of their own and their partner's aged parents.

2.3.4 Coping with competing demands

One important characteristic of students is how they regard competing demands for their time and energy. For HE students studying in Scottish FE, Lowe and Gayle (2007, p. 234) found they could not 'predict that certain categories of student would be more or less likely to achieve successful and stable integration of learning and life'. In the US, Nonis et al. (2006) found that students, with what appeared to be equivalent demands on their time, had different attitudes to and coped differently with those demands. Regardless, therefore, of inclination to expend effort on study, there is an issue of how students reason about competing demands and how they choose to resolve them.

The work of Houston and Rimmer (2007) and Donnelly *et al.* (2007) suggests that having expended one level of study effort, women might reduce effort but still optimise academic outcomes in subsequent semesters, suggesting one form of coping strategy. On the other hand, males might 'soldier on', making much the same study effort, despite earlier academic outcomes being indifferent.

2.3.5 Discipline, entry qualifications and persistence

There is considerable evidence that student academic grades vary by area of study. Yorke (2002) points out that in some disciplines the proportion of 'good degrees' (first class and upper seconds in the UK) is higher usually than in others. Houston *et al.* (2007) concluded that good grades tend to emerge more frequently in the same disciplines in the early undergraduate years. However, these effects are mediated by the entry qualifications of students. Interestingly, it is not necessarily traditional students who perform best. In universities in the UK and Australia, business students who took non-traditional routes to HE did better than those who proceeded directly from school to university (Donnelly *et al.*, 2007).

Further, the students who perform best in first level are not necessarily most likely to proceed with their studies. There are gender, age and ethnic dimensions to this (Houston *et al.*, 2007; Houston and Rimmer, 2008). Patrick (2001) and Leppel (2001) have suggested that other factors are relevant, such as student self-image, social perceptions, the professional or vocational ethos of studies and the mathematical intensity of a discipline. Thus persistence with studies is more likely among business, education or media students regardless of the quality of academic performances, because working in these areas fits with their self images and their perceptions of the social and vocational worth of such roles, and they appreciate studying modules that are not heavily mathematical.

However, what of those who do well academically in their disciplines but choose not to proceed with their studies? McInnes (2001) noted that student priorities are different today. Attaining good grades followed by progression to the next level of study may not be as high a priority for modern students as it was when their lecturers and tutors were students.

2.4 Institutional provision

The previous reasons for trading off work, life and study have concentrated on factors associated with student characteristics. However, institutions and the ways they structure and present programmes also have a role. It has long been recognised that student outcomes are affected by institutional factors (Tinto,

1975; Astin, 1984; Bean and Metzner, 1985). Further, there have been many changes to institutional provision over past decades. International moves to modularisation and semesterisation have been important. These are frequently seen as aspects of flexible provision, which are manifested in transformations and adjustments to the structure, administration and delivery of academic programmes (Murphy *et al.*, 2002).

2.4.1 Flexibility

Morgan-Klein (2003) described flexibility initiatives as:

- systemic (for example, the provision of part-time study routes, open learning and use of ICT);
- structural (for example, in the form of semesterisation);
- curricular (for example, degree of modularisation);
- pathway (exemplified by allowing accumulation of credit and its transfer between institutions);
- setting, meaning the diversity of institutions, sectors and the links between them in providing educational opportunities.

Even though flexibility is a global phenomenon (Morgan-Klein and Gray, 2000), there is evidence that it is not necessarily implemented in the interests of students. The main reasons for introducing some aspects of flexibility have been 'the personal ambitions of senior managers, pressure from external regulatory agencies and a desire to emulate initiatives undertaken by competitor institutions' (Morris, 2000, p. 239). Similarly, Cloonan (2004, p. 194) concluded that 'notions and practices of flexibility within higher education appear to be adopted for pragmatic rather than pedagogic reasons'.

2.4.2 Responding to flexibility

In terms of each student negotiating engagement with study, Morgan-Klein (2003) found that there is little appreciation of how students must flexibly accommodate work, family life, social activities and study. For example, to accommodate domestic life, employment and institutional constraints, such as the length of the teaching period, English university students reduced study load (Merrill, 2001; Bourgeois *et al.*, 1999). It is further possible that insistence on attendance at classes, or assuming students are able to attend classes, is also a hurdle to meaningful engagement given the multiple commitments of non-traditional students (Donnelly *et al.*, 2007).

In Scotland and Australia, female students exploited modular provision to reduce load in order to do as well as possible in those modules they attempted and/or to ensure they fulfilled rules on satisfactory progress (Donnelly *et al.*, 2007). This may have occurred at the expense of the coherence of their studies, the choice of modules to study and when to study them. On the other hand, it may have been a rational reaction to studying in environments where too many coursework assignments too frequently disrupted the rhythms of the rest of life.

Quality Assurance Agency (QAA) (2004) cite the case of students exploiting a rule designed to allow progression, even though a failure was recorded. Successive QAA audits, several external examiners and staff were concerned that the full range of learning outcomes were not attained, while students tactically avoided challenging modules. At another UK institution final degree awards were determined using an algorithm based on performances at each level of study. There was scope for students to 'play the system' by tactical withdrawal from some modules to avoid a lower classification, or not completing work as well as they might once a certain degree grade had been assured (Baty, 2005, p. 8). These examples reflect understandable responses to aspects of institutional provision.

2.4.3 Negotiating student engagement

Students who make these responses do not necessarily see the effects on their learning and the skills that they might not fully develop. This is not their fault. As McInnes (2001, p. 13) asserts, it is more useful for teaching and learning in practice 'to re-conceptualise the undergraduate experience as a process of negotiated engagement rather than assuming disengagement is an intractable problem and that students are to blame'. Further, on page 14 he wrote 'We are in urgent need of *creative* ideas to address the changing nature of student engagement' (italics added). Nonis *et al.* (2007, p. 30) referred to the need for students 'to re-evaluate how they spend their time' and that 'students view instructors as the most important component in their learning process, and as such, instructors can do a better job of communicating to students the importance of their own activities in the learning process'.

It was noted earlier that evidence from the US suggests that students have developed a sense of entitlement. It might be inferred that the imposition of fees in parts of the UK have generated a similar sense, because a number of universities have formulated 'contracts', which students are asked to sign, which point out that paying fees does not guarantee a degree will be awarded (Newman 2008, p. 14). A draft contract devised by the Universities and Colleges Law Network in the UK states 'it is a matter of the tuition fee giving access to teaching and other facilities, and of securing the opportunity to earn the degree by working diligently and consistently to meet the appropriate academic requirements' (ibid.).

Yet, even if this avoids litigation from unsuccessful students, it does not address the core issue of providing students with a creative means of engaging with study that fits with their own circumstances and helps them to negotiate a pathway to graduation via their own study effort, in other words via student-centred learning.

In making the photocopiable SAMI available, our intention is to provide assistance to instructors, lecturers and personal tutors in helping students to re-evaluate how they spend their time and in negotiating engagement with study. In the next section, the theoretical underpinnings of the SAMI are outlined.

3. THEORETICAL UNDERPINNINGS

The SAMI presented below draws on tools and theory from the following fields:

- learning styles and approaches to study;
- motivational interviewing and brief interventions;
- decision-making and problem-solving.

These are discussed next commencing with a review of learning styles and approaches to study.

3.1 Learning styles and approaches to study

The literature on interventions designed to aid learning and adopting particular approaches to it is a somewhat confusing and contradictory area. Some authors speak of learning styles, others of approaches to study. Some authors say these are unchangeable attributes while others claim they are changeable, depending on the learning environment.

There is a number of theories relating to how people learn. Four areas are generally recognised: behaviourist, cognitive, humanist and cultural approaches. Each has a different perspective on the way in which people learn and the resulting relationship with teaching. There is considerable interest in learning style, on the basis that recognition of approaches to learning by students and their teachers can improve student learning. It seems to be accepted generally that educational attainment depends not only on the nature of learning environments and students' abilities, but also on students' learning styles and the approaches they adopt to their studies. Some research focuses on the attributes of students, ignoring the context in which learning takes place. Other research focuses on learning techniques and environments while paying little attention to what students bring to the learning experience. Often, blame is attributed to the student or teacher. The wider context of learning, including national, international and institutional influences on students, is often overlooked.

Many studies (in looking at what students bring to learning) have considered learning styles and approaches to study, but frequently they have been beset by difficulties of definition, methodology and measurement.

In addition, studies which have aimed at improving study skills have been equivocal. Biggs (1988) concluded that appropriately contextualised study skills training with motivational support can work. However Ramsden *et al.* (1986) and Ramsden *et al.* (1987) note than in other circumstances such training may even be counter-productive. A similar finding relates to when study skills programmes are offered as adjuncts to the students' academic programme. The longer term impact, including the effect on transferability of skills to other subject areas, is inconclusive. See, for example, Gibbs (1997), Dansereau (1985) and Martin and Ramsden (1987).

Many theories of learning style have been devised. Coffield *et al.* (2004) reviewed 71 models, assigning each to a 'family' that was positioned on a continuum. Assignment to a family depended on 'the extent to which the authors of the model claim that styles are constitutionally based and relatively fixed, or believe that they are more flexible and open to change' (ibid., p. 9). The 'families' on the continuum are portrayed as:

- constitutionally based learning styles and preferences;
- cognitive structure;
- stable personality type;
- 'flexibly stable' learning preferences;
- learning approaches and strategies.

At one end of the continuum are 'those theorists with strong beliefs about the influence of genetics on fixed inherited traits and about the interaction of personality and cognition' (ibid., p. 10). At the other end of the continuum, 'theorists pay greater attention to personal factors such as motivation, and environmental factors like cooperative or individual learning' (op. cit.). Overall, the research field was found to be 'both extensive and conceptually confusing' (op. cit.).

Coffield *et al.* further undertook in-depth analysis of 13 widely used inventories developed to measure learning styles. They concluded that 'some of the best known and widely used instruments have such serious weaknesses (e.g. low reliability, poor validity and negligible impact on pedagogy) that we recommend that their use in research and in practice should be discontinued', while other more promising approaches should be researched further (ibid., p. 138).

Of the 13 inventories, only that of Allinson and Hayes (1996) was deemed satisfactory on each of four criteria – internal consistency, test-retest reliability, construct validity and predictive validity. However, this inventory was designed for and tested in organisational and business contexts, rather than in educational settings. The inventories of Apter *et al.* (1998) and Vermunt (1996) met three of the criteria in testing with students from seven different disciplines, studying either on-campus or in distance modes. According to Coffield *et al.*, Apter's model is a theory of personality rather than of learning styles, although the inventory was acknowledged as a useful addition to measures of learning style. Vermunt's inventory of learning styles could 'be safely used in higher education, both to assess approaches to learning reliably and validly, and to discuss with students changes in learning and teaching' (Coffield *et al.*, 2004, p. 138).

Inventories associated with Entwistle *et al.* (2000), Herrmann (1996) and Myers-Briggs (Myers and McCaulley, 1996) met two of the consistency and validity criteria. The other seven inventories performed badly and careful consideration should be given to whether or not they are used in academic settings (Coffield *et al.*, 2004). However, the Approaches and Study Skills Inventory for Students (ASSIST) associated with Entwistle, provides a 'sound basis for discussing effective and ineffective strategies for learning and for diagnosing students' approaches, orientations and strategies. It is an important aid for course design, curriculum and assessment design, including study skill support' (ibid., p. 138).

A condensed version of the ASSIST was evaluated as part of the development of the SAMI (Duffy, 2005; see also Tait and Entwistle, 1996; Duff, 1997; Entwistle *et al.*, 2000). This condensed ASSIST met all of the benchmarks applied in Coffield *et al.*'s analysis of 13 commonly used instruments. Consequently, it is concluded that the SAMI incorporates a reliable and valid tool appropriate to assess students' approaches to study.

3.2 Motivational interviewing

The Learning and Skills Development Agency (LSDA, 2003, p. 3) states that 'We know relatively little about what really motivates people to learn'. Following an extensive review of the educational literature, the Learning and Skills Research Centre (LSRC, 2004, p. 1) confirmed that 'Definitions of motivation are very rarely discussed in the literature, and the term is often invoked loosely, without definition, to explain why some learners progress while others do not'. Further, 'A key issue in defining "motivation" is the extent to which it is seen as an essentially internal individual character trait, or as a product of the interaction between individual and environment . . . particular social context and experience of educational process. Both interpretations can be found in the post-16 literature . . . sometimes used by the same author in the same article' (ibid., pp. 4–5).

Byrnes (2001, cited in LSRC, 2004, pp. 4–5) provides a standard definition of motivation as a 'construct that is used to explain the initiation, direction, intensity and persistence of an individual's behaviour in a particular situation'. This has been extended in LSRC (op. cit.) to include 'the notion of engagement, where the student is active, attentive, curious and willing to participate'. Often motivation is seen as 'intrinsic (a genuine desire to learn) or extrinsic (the pursuit of an external goal such as a qualification)' (op. cit.). Definitions are further confounded by Harlen and Crick (2003, p. 171) who state that 'The interaction of different aspects of motivation with a variety of personal characteristics mean that what motivates some students may alienate others'.

3.2.1 Theory and practice

The theory and practice of motivational interviewing has developed in areas where a change of behaviour is sought, such as seeking change in alcohol and drug use (Miller and Rollnick, 2002). Heather (2005) cites evidence in support of motivational interviewing that was gathered in a variety of settings and countries (Noonan and Moyers, 1997; Burke *et al.*, 2001; Dunn *et al.*, 2001; Burke *et al.*, 2002, p. 218). Lessons learned about successfully motivating individuals in these and other settings have been used in building the SAMI.

For Miller and Rollnick (2002, p. 25) 'Motivational interviewing is a client-centred, directive method for enhancing intrinsic motivation to change by exploring and resolving ambivalence'. Ambivalence or dissonance is '. . . a discrepancy between the present state of affairs and how one wants it to be . . . Discrepancy may be triggered by an awareness of and discontent with the costs of one's present course of behaviour and by perceived advantages of behaviour change. When a behaviour is seen as conflicting with important personal goals (such as one's health, success, family happiness, or positive image), change is more likely to occur' (ibid., p. 38). They note that motivational interviewing is more focussed and goal directed than non-directive counselling, with the counsellor being 'intentionally directive in' resolving ambivalence (op. cit.).

Rollnick and Miller (1995) presented seven points that, for them, characterise the 'spirit of motivational interviewing'.

1 Motivation to change is elicited from the individual. Instead of coercion, confrontation or external imposition, motivational interviewers try to identify and mobilise an individual's internal values and aims with a view to stimulating change in behaviour.

2 In motivational interviewing the role of the counsellor is to elicit an individual's *own* expression of their ambivalence; and then to provide support while the client identifies ways that would resolve the ambivalence, bring about change and be recognised by the client as an acceptable way forward. By contrast, in other forms of intervention, the counsellor's role is to articulate and resolve an individual's ambivalence or dissonance.

3 In motivational interviewing direct persuasion by the counsellor is avoided, as this may induce resistance from an individual and make it difficult for the person to accept that change is possible, appropriate and carries benefits that are worth the effort of changing behaviour.

4 Compared with many counselling approaches, motivational interviewing is quiet and eliciting, rather than aggressive, confrontational or argumentative, which may push individuals towards inappropriate changes in their behaviour.

5 A counsellor using motivational interviewing would aim to 'elicit, clarify and resolve ambivalence in a client-centred and respectful counseling atmosphere' (Rollnick and Miller, 1995, p. 328). Examining ambivalence and resolving it are key.

6 Readiness to change is not an internal trait of an individual, but is instead explained as a 'fluctuating product of interpersonal interaction' (ibid., p. 329).

7 Instead of an expert/recipient relationship (which often gives power and control to the counsellor) the relationship within motivational interviewing is more one of 'partnerships or companionship' in which there is respect for the autonomy and freedom of choice of the individual in deciding to change, or not to change.

Rollnick and Miller do not perceive motivational interviewing as a set of techniques that counsellors apply to or use on their clients. Rather, it is a 'subtle balance of directive and client-centred components, shaped by a guiding philosophy and understanding of what triggers change' (ibid., p. 329). The approach is often combined with the methods of decision-making and goal-setting to enhance confidence in bringing about a change in behaviour. Further, brainstorming (applied in decision-making and problem-solving approaches) can assist an individual to be more creative in identifying how change can be achieved. With increased confidence that change is possible, with increased creativity in deciding on possible change strategies, and with ownership of the recognition of ambivalence and how to resolve it, individuals can prepare personal change – plans which are meaningful to them. These elements permit individuals to move from being concerned about their behaviour to taking action to resolve this concern or ambivalence.

3.3 Making decisions about study habits

In terms of value for money, Coffield *et al.* (2004) challenged proponents of learning styles to do better than researchers in other areas that compete for government funding, such as formal assessment and metacognition. In designing the SAMI, a version of analytical decision-making (see below), is employed to analyse current study patterns and lead students to plan change and evaluate their progress. Thus, the SAMI draws on both metacognitive- and learning-style approaches. Commenting on the largest meta-analysis of research conducted on educational instruction by Marzano (1998), Coffield *et al.* (2004, p. 136) concluded 'that approaches which were directed at the metacognitive level of setting goals, choosing appropriate strategies and monitoring progress are more effective in improving knowledge outcomes than those which simply aim to engage learners at the level of presenting information for understanding and use'.

Some authors divide the analytical technique of reaching decisions and resolving problems into four key steps or stages (Whetten and Cameron, 2002), while others advocate more. Adair (1985; 1997) distinguished five or seven steps. Based on one of the current author's experiences in counselling, it was decided to model the decision-making sections of the SAMI as follows:

- stage 1: orientate yourself;
- stage 2: define the issue;
- stage 3: generate alternatives;
- stage 4: evaluate alternatives and make a decision;
- stage 5: set goals, make a plan and implement;
- stage 6: evaluate and monitor.

3.3.1 Stage 1: orientate yourself

Orientation has been set out as the initial step in counselling implementations (D'Zurrilla and Goldfried, 1971). Frequently, people feel strongly or are emotional about issues that could require change and about the change process itself. This can make it seem that some issues cannot be resolved. It is important therefore to attempt to stand back and be objective. One common approach to attaining detachment is to think that an issue faced by an individual is not their problem, but is an area where a colleague or friend must make a decision. By doing so, an individual may examine their own views of the benefits of the current situation and of change.

A similar concern is the need to differentiate between fact and fiction and to identify objective information (Whetten and Cameron, 2002). They also refer to the need to identify clearly what expectation or standard is being violated in the current situation. Adair (1985) drew attention to becoming aware of signs of a problem arising. Nevertheless the message at this point is clear: attempt to be objective. For example, a student considering a change of study approach may be anxious about the impact of a different study regime on their capacity to work, whether it is to maintain life or lifestyle (see Section 2 of the main text, page 2). Overcoming this worry can be difficult; not doing so could mean that the student is unable to be objective enough to see that they may not need to study for longer periods, but might need simply to study at different times.

3.3.2 Stage 2: define the issue

It is important to clarify exactly what is to be resolved. Further, it is important to focus on one situation at a time rather than wide-ranging unclear difficulties. This clarity of definition can be difficult to attain. It is often easier to describe difficulties in vague terms, but this is unhelpful as the wrong issue may be addressed or the real problem may be avoided. To say, for example, that 'my approach to study is not good' is vague. It might suggest that there is a problem with the student's motivation to study; it might avoid the issue of having little free time. Problem definitions and statements of aims and objectives need to be specific. Chang and Kelly (1993) suggest that an aid to obtaining a precise definition is to state the issue by beginning with the word 'How'. Rather than say that 'My approach to study is not good', it may be better to say, 'How can I improve my approach to study?' Even more specifically, the issue may be 'How can I manage my time better?' Rather than say that 'Relations with students in my group for coursework are strained', it may be more useful to say 'How can I improve relations with students in my group?' As a lecturer in FE or HE the issue may be 'How can I motivate students to improve their approaches to study?'

Before moving on to the next stage, it is imperative that the issue is accurately and unambiguously specified. If not, the solutions generated may not resolve the problem under consideration. Writing about problem-solving in a management context, Whetten and Cameron (2002, p. 162) concluded that 'managers often propose a solution before an adequate definition of a problem has been given. This may lead to solving the "wrong" problem. The definition step in problem-solving, therefore, is extremely important'. Adair (1997, p. 22), more informally asked 'Are you clear about what you are trying to do? Where are you now and where do you want to get to?' Further, it is possible that giving only slight consideration to this stage could mean that a definition may be cast in the form of a disguised solution. For example, 'The problem is that I need to study every Thursday evening' rather than 'How can I study and have time for other activities?'

Another factor given by Whetten and Cameron (2002, p.161) is relevant to the situation of students who are considering changing their study patterns and approaches. They recommend 'all individuals are tapped as information sources'. This could mean talking about study habits with friends, relatives and contacts at college or university.

3.3.3 Stage 3: generate alternatives

Having identified an issue to resolve, next generate a range of possible solutions. 'Much research on problem solving (e.g., March, 1999) supports the prescription that the quality of solutions can be significantly enhanced by considering multiple alternatives' (Whetten and Cameron, 2002, p. 162). This process is often easy in a small group as an idea suggested by one person may trigger another idea from someone else. However, a person could conduct this stage without assistance.

It is important not to evaluate ideas as they are suggested but, rather, record them for later consideration. Evaluating as you go will slow down the process of generating solutions, prevent creative suggestions being made or prevent others building on earlier notions. It is important that no criticism is made of suggestions at this stage as again this will inhibit the flow of possible solutions.

All suggestions should therefore be written down no matter how strange they may appear at first. Evaluating early or as new alternatives are devised may rule out optimal solutions. The maxim is 'Many alternative solutions should be produced before any of them are evaluated' (Whetten and Cameron, 2002, p. 162). The aim is to generate many options on the basis that quantity breeds quality. Some authors suggest ten or more options should be produced; Adair (1997) suggests that at least three or four are devised. In the context of students with busy lives, 'at least three or four' should be accomplished easily in a short period of reflection.

If a mature student with a job and a family defines their problem as how to obtain sufficient marks to ensure that they are able to re-enrol, then some brainstorming suggestions might be:

drop non-core subjects;

prepare an appeal against an adverse examination-board decision now;

do not attempt coursework assessments in non-core subjects;

ask family members to do domestic tasks when examinations and courseworks are due;

take annual leave from work to concentrate on assessments;

send the family away to remove distractions;

go away and become a study hermit during crucial assessment periods;

study non-core subjects only when tired;

study only non-core subjects on the train;

give up work and depend on partner's income and a personal loan;

visit the college or university study skills laboratory;

employ specialist tutors for core subjects;

employ a study coach or counsellor;

work part time.

3.3.4 Stage 4: evaluate alternatives and make a decision

In this stage, assess and compare the advantages and disadvantages of alternative solutions, bearing in mind the definition from Stage 2. That is, remember what is to be resolved and consider the likely consequences, short- and long-term, of each alternative solution.

Now delete poor options. Before doing so, identify what is meant by the term 'poor'. This may involve evaluation of possible solutions against a standard. Some (for example, Whetten and Cameron, 2002) suggest that clear guidelines are identified to assist in rejecting and selecting options from the list. Consider the case of a young student enrolled for the first time at college or university, who works part-time and enjoys many leisure activities. The issue this student defines might be the same as the one defined by the mature student considered above: 'How can I earn enough marks to ensure that I can re-enrol?' Some alternative solutions might be:

work less;

reduce the number of courseworks and examinations attempted;

cut back on social engagements;

study every work-day evening between 7.00 and 10.00;

don't visit the coffee shop on campus;

attend more lectures and tutorials;

give up work;

move back to parents' home;

play less sport;

work in library while at college or university;

employ specialist tutors;

learn to manage time.

This student might opt to make their selection of preferred solution on the basis of the following criteria:

I   risk;
II   effort;
III   income;
IV   reputation.

Consequently, the student may assess returning to the parental home in the following ways:

I   a risk to social life, because they would no longer be able to have parties as often as in the past;
II   they would not have to worry about shopping, cooking, cleaning and managing a household budget, so more effort could be applied to study;
III   less or none of the student's income would be required to pay bills;
IV   by withdrawing to their parents' home and studying more, the student may fear gathering a reputation in their social circle for being a swot or being unable to cope alone, while on the other hand realising that their standing with lecturers and tutors could rise.

This and similar reasoning would allow the student to put a line through those options which are rejected as poor in the list of alternative solutions. The remaining options would then be considered and compared, by weighing up the advantages and disadvantages of each. Thus, the student might reject the option of not working at all as poor. However, while the alternative of moving back to their parents may evaluate as being risky and having undesirable reputational consequences, it may be preferable (less poor) compared with the drain on their income of alternatives of employing specialist tutors or the reputational consequences of playing less sport.

Before progressing to the next stage, preferred solutions are prioritised. If using a flipchart or other paper record, this can be accomplished by simply placing the number '1' beside the first preferred option, the number '2' beside the second preferred option and so on.

3.3.5 Stage 5: set goals, make a plan and implement

Once a preferred solution has been identified, desired outcomes should be set and a plan made to implement the solution. Measurable, realistic and achievable outcomes are required to ensure that progress on the issue defined in Stage 2 is recognised and that in the final stage (below), progress can be monitored and the preferred solution evaluated. This is sometimes paraphrased as 'if you don't know where you're going, you won't know when you've arrived'.

In the case of the young student wanting to ensure that they can re-enrol, possible goals might be:

1 attain A grades in each subject;
2 attain passes in each assessment and be allowed to progress to the next level of study;
3 attain passes in core subjects only and be allowed to enrol in some modules at the next level and in those that were not passed at the lower level;
4 attain passes so as to enable enrolment in all relevant modules at the next level while carrying one or two at the lower level;
5 aim to be enrolled next only in modules that were not passed.

These are distinct outcomes and can be assessed when final marks and examination-board decisions become available. Also, it is prudent to set goals that can be assessed to evaluate a course of action as a semester unfolds. For example:

6 pass each coursework and each examination in each semester;
7 pass coursework in only core areas and examinations in each module.

Whetten and Cameron (2002) suggest that the strategy of 'small wins' (Weick, 1984) is a sound approach to implementation. In this, solutions are implemented little by little and the outcomes made public. Thus, for example, students who decide their preferred option is to return to the parental home, might first discuss this decision with their parents and with current flatmates to get agreement that the solution is feasible. Next, the students might set a timetable, spanning say a month, in which they actually move away from their current accommodation and return to their parents. This might be made known to lecturers and tutors, so that they too understand that a new approach to study is to be expected.

Following this, small wins in the form of passing coursework assignments and tests should be publicised, providing affirmation to family, friends, former housemates and academic staff that the solution is effective. According to Whetten and Cameron (2002) this ensures buy-in by those involved (say in the form of acceptance by parents and former housemates that moving back home has been worth any disruption caused to them) and it generates a sense of progress being made. Further, telling others who are involved that small wins are being attained, promotes student persistence and perseverance.

3.3.6 Stage 6: evaluate and monitor

With appropriate goals, it is possible to evaluate success in terms of the definition set out in Stage 2. Assuming that realistic goals are set within agreed timeframes, then these may be reviewed to evaluate and monitor the success of the preferred solution. If goals are not achieved, then it is possible to reflect on why not and revise the action plan accordingly. If goals are achieved then there is immediate recognition that progress has been made. Further, faced with another decision to take about study, students will have greater confidence that they can apply the decision-making technique to bring about effective change.

In the case of the young student wanting to ensure that re-enrolment is possible, the seven goals given above are linked to the problem definition; two of them (6 and 7), in that they relate to coursework, relate to timeframes which are shorter than a semester (about a few weeks usually), while the others have timeframes in which some outcomes can be assessed at each examination diet.

Another point to note is that outcomes may be 'manifest' or 'latent' (Adair, 1997). The former are consequences that can be foreseen potentially, while the probability of observing the latter, unintended consequences is low. Should unintended consequences have substantial effects, this suggests that another round of the six stages is required. For example, should the student find that moving back to the parental home imposes additional unexpected costs for travel to work and to place of study – either money (because fares rise or the car breaks down) or time (because of roadworks causing delays for long periods or because bus timetables change) – the student could re-visit the decision-making process.

3.4 Brief Intervention

In the previous three sub-sections, the literature on learning styles, motivational interviewing and decision-making was considered. It is possible to incorporate tools from these theoretical perspectives into an instrument which students can use to consider changes to their study approaches. In many cases, people change their behaviour without formal treatment. For example, people reduce their alcohol consumption without formal assistance. Many people go on diets and lose weight without attending diet clinics or support groups. Others give up smoking without seeing a counsellor for assistance. The stages of change for those attending treatment and those not attending seem to be the same. 'Treatment can be thought of as facilitating what is a natural process of change' (Miller and Rollnick, 2002, p. 4). Further, many people change with only a little assistance from the helping professions, as opposed to longer-term treatment interventions. Miller and Rollnick report, 'The fascinating point is that so much change occurs after so little counseling' (ibid., p.5).

Many types of brief or minimal interventions are used in helping people make changes in their lives. In his review of brief interventions and their role in relation to more intensive treatment of alcohol problems, Duffy (1994, p. 4) outlines the nature of minimal interventions. 'Many studies describe "brief" as being only one interview, others a series of interviews, others still offering a self-help manual with little or even no personal contact.' Key elements of a brief intervention are captured in FRAMES, a conceptual framework developed by Bien *et al.* (1993):

F   FEEDBACK on assessment results;
R   RESPONSIBILITY – changing is up to the client;
A   ADVICE to reduce or stop problematic behaviour;
M   MENU of options in the process of change;
E   EMPATHY features in most descriptions in some form, although some appear confrontational;
S   SELF-EFFICACY is promoted to reduce feelings of helplessness and increase empowerment to undertake change.

Brief interventions aimed at assisting people to change their behaviour have been evaluated across a range of professional areas. In the field of alcohol counselling, the benefits of brief interventions have been assessed in controlled studies. Reduction in alcohol use and related problems were identified following a minimal intervention. The conclusion is that 'Minimal interventions, assuming they are well planned and executed, can have quite an impact, often as significant as that offered by more extensive intervention' (Duffy 1994, p .4).

4. THE DESIGN OF THE INSTRUMENT

The SAMI was developed in line with theory relating to learning styles, motivational interviewing and decision-making. It was designed to raise awareness of approaches to study, to increase ambivalence about change and to encourage students to set achievable goals and implement change plans. Recall that evidence from other areas (such as reducing difficulties related to the misuse of alcohol or drugs) confirms that often people can make changes without intensive interventions. The SAMI was specifically designed for this study as a brief intervention in line with Miller and Rollnick's theory of motivational interviewing. In the following sub-sections the instrument is discussed as follows:

- awareness, dissonance or ambivalence raising (see Sub-sections 4.1.1 and 4.1.2);
- self-review of the advantages and disadvantages of change (Sub-section 4.2);
- analytical decision-making to find ways of dealing with study problems (Sub-section 4.3).

Excerpts from the SAMI are reproduced within this section and examples of students' responses gathered in the study of Duffy (2005) are also provided. The whole instrument is given as a photocopiable resource in Appendix 1 on page 51.

4.1 Exploring ambivalence

4.1.1 Self-rating of actual and potential performance

Immediately following the cover page of the instrument, students are drawn to reflect on the likely outcomes of their study habits, via the statement:

> This booklet has been prepared to help you in any decisions you may make about your studying. After you have filled it in, you may find it useful to refer to it from time to time. The first thing is to consider how well you are doing with your study at the moment.

The intention at this early point is to make students aware that it is they who are responsible for their study and their academic outcomes. This is followed by three items that explore feelings of ambivalence about study approach. The tone of the wording in the statement above is intended to be non-threatening, consistent with Miller and Rollnick (2002). The use of the word 'you' puts each student in the role of decision-maker. The use of the word 'any' in the first line of the statement is intended to cover the possibility that students have the option of deciding not to change their study habits (ibid.). In this way, students who decide to continue as before, simply do so. For example, some mature students with significant external obligations might have felt they are already studying as well as they can. This reflects the 'equipoise' notion, where the counsellor creates an environment in which the client has control over the decision to change or not (Miller and Rollnick, 2002, p. 91).

The two questions in 1.1 explore perceptions of current and potential performance. The third question (1.2) explores whether different responses in 1.1 are causes for concern and if so what is of concern. This is the first question posed in 1.1.

1.1

> On a score from 1-9, how well do think you are doing with your study (where 1 is 'not very well' and 9 is 'very well')? Place an X in the box below the appropriate number.

Not very well   Very well

1	2	3	4	5	6	7	8	9

A scale is provided which students use to indicate one of nine possible ratings. The lowest of these is Value 1, described as 'not very well'; the highest is Value 9, described as 'very well' (capturing excellence and coping well). The first item on the SAMI is referred to as the 'How well' question.

This question is drawn from the ASSIST questionnaire. Tait and Entwistle (1996) found that responses to it were predictors of academic achievement. In the SAMI, it sets the scene by asking each student to reflect on their study patterns and approaches, rather than relying on external feedback from tutors and marks on assignments and examinations. The intention is to introduce self-review, a key aspect of motivational interviewing (Miller and Rollnick, 2002).

The next item in 1.1, referred to as the 'Potential' question, is directed to students' perceptions of what might be possible.

On a score from 1-9, how well do think you could score if you really tried your best (where 1 is 'not very well' and 9 is 'very well')? Place an X in the box below the appropriate number.

Not very well   Very well

1	2	3	4	5	6	7	8	9

The intention is to generate a degree of ambivalence or cognitive dissonance if there is a difference between the responses to this question and the previous one. Within motivational interviewing, exploring ambivalence is recognised as being an important aspect of assisting the process of change. For example, if a score of three was identified for the question on current performance and a score of eight on potential performance, students might feel a degree of ambivalence: their expected actual score is low, while their potential score is high. Becoming aware of this dissonance may serve to increase a student's awareness of the need to change their approach to study.

The exploration of dissonance is continued in SAMI Question 1.2, where students are asked if a difference in their 'How well' and 'Potential' scores is worthy of comment or consideration. As shown on p. 24, a box is provided in which to write a response. Some examples of statements from students are included. In brackets are the students' 'How well' score followed by their 'Potential' score. Where concern is expressed because a difference exists, this might indicate students who are contemplating or would contemplate change. These are known as 'contemplators of change' in the literature. Those students whose responses to the 'How well' and 'Potential' questions are the same, but who desire an improved rating on the 'Potential' question (and presumably, improved academic outcome) may also be change contemplators.

1.2	If the above scores differ, in what way does this bother you (if at all)?
A.	It shows that I am not doing my best and I will therefore have a lower chance to succeed (6/9).
	I don't think I am studying as hard as I should be (5/7).
	It shows I need to put more effort to study more (7/9).
	It bothers me, as I am not doing my best at this particular time (6/8).
	I realise I should be trying harder, but when working full time and having family commitments it is very difficult (6/8).

Another group is distinguished in the literature. Those who are 'not bothered', that is those who recorded a difference between 'How well' and 'Potential' scores but do not think this is a bother. These may be students who are not contemplating change. They are referred to as 'pre-contemplators of change'.

This section of the SAMI necessarily precedes the next, as the intention is to lead participants to first acknowledge they are ambivalent about study approaches, if this is the case.

4.1.2 Reflection on approach to study (self-administration of the condensed ASSIST)

The questions in Section 2 of the SAMI are intended to raise awareness about students' approaches to study. To begin with, awareness or ambivalence engendered in earlier items is further increased by inviting subjects to complete the 20 questions of the condensed ASSIST. Students scored themselves from one to five on each statement corresponding to disagreement (1) through to agreement (5). The 20 statements consist of ten to assess a student's deep approach to learning and ten designed to assess the student's strategic approach to study. For example, the statement 'It's important to me to be able to follow the argument or see the reasoning behind something' is one of the deep items; and the statement 'I generally try to make good use of my time during the day' is a strategic item.

Immediately following the condensed ASSIST (2.1 of the SAMI), students are told about typical scores and about the possibility of a link between scores and actual academic performance (such a link was found in a pilot conducted by Duffy (2005)). The intention is to stir participants to undertake a self-review of their condensed ASSIST score relative to the scores of others, on average, who have completed the instrument. To initiate this reflection, respondents were provided with space in which to record their total scores. On one hand, if they appeared to be performing relatively well, they may see little need to change behaviour. On the other hand, if they were not performing well, they may be more inclined to make changes.

The inclusion of the condensed ASSIST was intended to promote another layer of thinking about study. To this end students are next asked what they like or dislike about their total condensed ASSIST scores. The intention is that students will probe concerns they may have about their scores. Students were then asked the question (2.2) in the following dialogue box. Student responses are shown, together with condensed ASSIST scores in parentheses. Note that students with scores over 90 seemed to be more than happy with their totals. By contrast, one student with a score of 77 was a change contemplator (see Section 3 of the main text, pages 12–13), while another student in the box below with the same score may not have been contemplating change. Overall, there seems to be a direct link between total score and realisation that change should be considered.

2.2	What do you like/dislike about your total score for the above questions?
A.	I liked how my score was (95).
	I am proud of my score (94).
	It is reasonably good but there is still room for improvement (80).
	It could probably be better if I put more effort in (77).
	I though it was an all right score (77).
	It is quite high but could be higher (72).
	My score is not good enough – more effort is needed (71).
	Made me realise I should do more so as to achieve more. I'm not doing my best (67).

Up to this point (that is, up to 2.2 in the SAMI), students are encouraged to become aware of any concerns they may have about their study approaches.

4.2 Decisional balance

In Section 3 of the SAMI, the items labelled 3.1–3.12 invite students to look more closely at their study behaviour and their aims. The intention is to elicit 'self-motivational statements' or 'change talk'. Motivational interviewing encourages reflection on the costs and benefits of two elements:

1 continuing with the current study regime;
2 changing the approach to study.

Element 1 is considered in items 3.1–3.6.

4.2.1 Costs and benefits of maintaining the *status quo*

Current study issues

The specific intention of item 3.1 is to allow students to express their concerns about current difficulties they may be experiencing with study. In face-to-face motivational interviewing this question is phrased so that respondents can state their *own* concerns. In this self-administered setting, the student is not led by an interviewer. Rather, the intention is that each student will think seriously about problems and write them down.

3.1	The problems I have with my approach to studying are:
A.	Not enough time. I usually get interrupted and distracted.
	I need peace and quiet when studying, and that is not always possible.
	I just can't get into a routine of fitting everything else in my life around studying.
	I feel I need to focus more and spend more time studying.
	I work full time, have family commitments and so time management skills in my approach to studying is very important.

From the responses shown, it is clear that some students took this opportunity to set out a range of difficulties, such as time management, being easily interrupted and needing peace and quiet. For some, the responses were vague, as in 'I feel I need to focus more' and 'I just can't get into a routine'. While students recorded numerous difficulties, it does not imply that they are concerned about the issues or that they intend to change to alleviate the problems. This is explored in the following items.

Concern over difficulties with current approach

In motivational interviewing, the aim is not simply to list difficulties experienced, but to elicit concern about them. Thus, the next item (3.2) provides an opportunity for this by asking what it is that worries the individual about the difficulties they have listed. An example of this might be a concern about eating chocolate biscuits, which might be expressed as: 'I am worried that my excessive weight will cause me health problems'. The concern is not about putting on weight now, but rather about the potential for longer-term health difficulties if excessive consumption of chocolate biscuits continues.

3.2	What is it that worries you about these difficulties?
A.	My only worry is that I will not be able to change this and that I will not do as well as I want to.
	That I might fail my assignments.
	That I don't put enough effort in and fail to get good grades.
	That I won't do as well and that I'll fail and not graduate.
	I worry about not being successful in the course, or scoring low grades.

An example which relates directly to study is provided by the student who responded to item 3.2 with the statement 'I might fail my assignments'. If probed about why this is of concern, the student might add that, 'I'll fail and not graduate'. If this were the case, it is the possibility of not graduating that is the ultimate concern, not failing assignments. Of course, not graduating could induce other problems, such as not finding the preferred type of job, missing promotion or suffering reduced self-esteem.

Benefits of current approach

Next (in item 3.3) participants are asked to reflect on the other side of the decisional balance, which is to identify the benefits of maintaining the *status quo*. This not only allows the individual to start looking at both costs and benefits of change, it is likely to give the student the feeling that the SAMI is a detached document. In this sense it can be said to conform to Miller and Rollnick's (2002, p. 91) sense of 'equipoise'.

3.3	If I continue to study in the way I do now, the benefits would be:
A.	I 'might' pass but my chances are lower.
	Not a lot. I need to improve my study routine.
	This would not be very beneficial because I need to study more to reach my aim – to pass this course.
	To continue with my studies ensuring that my other commitments are met i.e. kids and work.
	I could scrape through the degree. I can prove to myself that it can be done and I suppose I may feel quite happy with that.

The next question (item 3.4) also relates to the benefits of maintaining the *status quo* and not changing.

3.4	In what way are these aspects beneficial to you?
A.	They are beneficial as I hope to learn new aspects to help me become a good nurse.
	I hopefully will pass my assignments.
	To pass the module means bringing me closer to my degree, and hopefully what I have learned I will be able to use in my nursing practice.
	Writing about my concerns will encourage me to organise myself better.
	Personal goals would be achieved. Academic qualifications obtained.

The point raised here is that individuals should be aware of what might be lost if they make a change. If they make a change and then discover that they have lost something important to them (and didn't realise they would lose it), then the change process may not last. This could be because what is lost is more important than what is to be gained by the change.

Drawbacks if the current approach is maintained

Next students are invited to identify drawbacks if they maintain their current study activities.

3.5	If I continue to study in the way I do now, the drawbacks would be:
A.	I would fail for not studying enough. If I do not stick to studying when I say, I might not finish the course. I may not be able to take enough information in. I know I need to start devoting more designated time to have enough info to help me. I'll be cramming at the end of the module and not giving my best effort due to lack of time.

Change talk is again stimulated when, in item 3.6, students express concerns about drawbacks they have with maintaining the *status quo*.

3.6	What is it that particularly concerns you about these drawbacks?
A.	It could be my last chance at this course. That I will not have as much understanding as others in my cohort. I want to pass them and I would be disappointed if I didn't pass. Failing and knowing that I could have done better. That I may not be putting my best into it.

Taken together, items 3.1–3.6 reflect two important features of motivational interviewing. First, students should not simply list difficulties or advantages, but should be drawn to consider why they are regarded as such (Miller and Rollnick, 2002). In 3.1–3.6, students have been invited to do this for their current study approaches. Second, students are encouraged to make links between their behaviour and consequent difficulties. This can be seen by comparing the flow from item 3.1 where participants are invited to consider 'problems' to item 3.3 when they think about 'benefits', and then on to item 3.5 to consider 'drawbacks'. The intention is to elicit *concern*, not just the identification of a problem (Miller and Rollnick, 2002).

4.2.2 Costs and benefits of change

Drawbacks of changing approach

In items 3.7 to 3.12 that follow, students are asked to contemplate ambivalence about potential changes in their study approaches. In item 3.7 students are prompted to list drawbacks; then in item 3.8 they are invited to reflect on them.

3.7	If I changed my approach to studying, the drawbacks would be:
A.	I will have to cut out some of my other activities. Less time socialising! Not socialising as much as I do. Would I have enough time to do my other activities? Less time with my family. Family life would suffer, and at the end of the day, my family comes first. I would feel selfish and guilty devoting time to something that only concerns me.

3.8	What is it that particularly concerns you about these drawbacks?
A.	I may not be able to do everything. I am particularly concerned about lack of time. Failing my assignment. Not achieving my own goals and expectations. Not achieving my optimal score. Less leisure time, loss of hobbies.

Benefits of changing approach

Having identified negative consequences in 3.7 and 3.8, students were given the opportunity to explore the benefits of change. The following item (3.9) provides a further opportunity for change talk, or self-motivational statements. The question is deliberately worded as 'If I changed...', with the emphasis on 'I'. This is likely to elicit a statement beginning with 'I', such as 'I would be able to get a higher grade'. There is no single mirror image of item 3.8. Rather, this is more fully explored in the next three items that provide a means for respondents to define the main problem they have with their current approach to study. This is later taken up as the subject of a self-administered decision-making session.

3.9	If I changed my approach to studying, the benefits would be:
A.	More organised, more time to complete assignments and collect information.
	I may produce work which is structured more clearly.
	I would submit a better piece of work, hence get a better mark.
	Possibly less pressure in last 2–3 weeks.
	I would get all the study done at ease and then not be worried about falling behind.
	I would be organised in my approach.
	More time in achieving goals expectations. Financial benefit.
	I would reach my full potential, knowing I put my best in to it.

Defining the issue (Step 2 in analytical decision-making)

First with item 3.10, each student's attention is focussed on the obstacles they see in bringing about change. Note the emphasis on the student via the use of the words 'me' and 'my' in the question posed in this item.

3.10	What are the main obstacles to me changing my approach to studying?
A.	Changing my social life.
	Need to work for money. Need to spend time with family and loved ones.
	Work, finance, family commitments.
	Time, work commitments.
	Not enough quality study time. Work 9-5, have a child.

In responding to the next item (3.11) students would reflect on and summarise why they wish to change. In face-to-face counselling, the counsellor may provide this 'recap'. In the SAMI, individuals are invited to provide this summary themselves. To elicit talk of personal change, the word 'I' is used, as was the case in earlier questions.

3.11	The reasons I have for changing my approach to study are:
A.	So that I can pass my assignments and feel happier within myself.
	To gain better results. Self-esteem.
	Coping better would have a beneficial effect on my life in general – and hopefully on my studies in particular.
	The reason for me changing my approach is to make study more relaxed and less all-consuming. Ensuring that I allocate time for all aspects of my life.
	To help me achieve my goal of gaining the qualification I am aiming for and also to gain a good knowledge base for practice.

This approach is continued in the next item of the SAMI, where students are invited to clearly define the main problem with their current approach to study (see Section 3 of the main text, pages 14–15). They are asked to be specific. The aim is to elicit a problem definition (see Section 3 as above) that will be the basis for the next stage of the SAMI.

3.12	So what really is the main problem in relation to your approach to study? Be very, very specific.
A.	Time management and prioritising my tasks with social life.
	Not enough time to study on a daily basis, due to other commitments that are just as important to me.
	I'm quite content to be a 'B' student if it means compromising family commitments. So my main problem is time.
	Time allocation. Work-load. Personal aspects, family and full time job and study.
	I feel perhaps I have to complete my degree rather than want to. I have started, so I have to finish.

What follows next in the SAMI are questions and statements aimed at leading each student to apply analytical decision-making to the issue of changing study approach.

4.3 Resolving decisional imbalance

4.3.1 Generate alternatives (Step 3 of analytical problem-solving)

As it is thought that 'quantity breeds quality' in brainstorming, students are encouraged to generate up to ten possible alternative solutions to the main problem defined in item 3.12. Item 4.1, reproduced from the SAMI on p. 34, contains some solutions identified by students, with the student's problem definition shown in parentheses.

4.1

Now have another look at your answer to Question 3.12. Stand back and try to be objective. Try to list as many possible ways of resolving this problem (around 10 ideas).			

Solutions	Please write in this column what you think may be a possible solution to what you have identified as your main problem. Ignore the two columns on the right for a minute, you will be asked to consider these shortly.	Delete	Prioritise
Solution 1	Set aside extra time for study (Find time to research subject.)		
Solution 2	Decrease working hours/give up one of my days off. (Not enough time to study on a daily basis.)		
Solution 3	Go to a quiet place to study/set up study area/study in library. (Too much else going on. Other people requiring my attention.)		
Solution 4	Take annual leave. (Too much else going on. Other people requiring my attention.)		
Solution 5	Make up a study timetable/improve time management skills. (Time management.)		

Solution 6	Read more on the train. (Problem is time.)		
Solution 7	Get up an hour earlier/work through the night/study for short periods of time after work. (Problem is time.)		
Solution 8	Obtain study time from employer. (Problem is time.)		
Solution 9	Give my husband more household tasks – ironing. Seek family support. (Time management.)		
Solution 10	Home in on the assignment/do not over read. Difficulty is just look at it as a means to an end. (Recognise the assignment as the important part.)		

4.3.2 Evaluate alternatives and make a decision (Stage 4 of decision-making)

> Now read again the main problem you are trying to resolve. Bearing this in mind, get rid of the poor options.
> Place an 'x' in the 'Delete' column above to identify solutions you want to get rid of.

First students use the third column of item 4.1 to denote those options that are considered poor or unworkable. Next students identify and prioritise (using column 4 of 4.1) what they believe are the most appropriate/relevant solutions for them. This is prompted with the statements:

> In the 'Prioritise' column above:
>
> Mark with a 1 the solution you think is most appropriate/relevant.
> Mark with a 2 the solution you think is the next most appropriate/relevant.
> Mark with a 3 the next most appropriate/relevant.

4.3.3 Set goals, make a plan and implement (Stage 5 of decision-making)

So far, students have been in control of problem definition and their roles as decision makers are maintained throughout the completion of item 4.1, including what changes, if any, they plan to make. This continues in the next three items of the SAMI (item 4.2.1 below is an example), where students consider how they could put the three most highly prioritised solutions into effect 'in a realistic and achievable manner'. They are asked specifically to develop a plan for each by completing the sentence 'I will put this into action by ...' At this stage too, control of potential change remains with the student.

4.2.1	How can you put this solution into action in a realistic and achievable manner? Develop a plan by completing the following sentence:
A.	I will put this into action by ...
	Going to the library to study, instead of the house with less distractions.
	Complete the literature search by 31st March by browsing a minimum of two articles per week.
	Creating a study area at home.
	Marking on the family calendar when I will be unavailable due to study time.
	Realistically setting out a study programme and adhering to it strictly.
	Negotiating with my wife possible times to study in the library.
	Allocating time more.
	Sitting down and listing work commitments/other commitments and highlight the best times to complete my studies.
	Seeking guidance from the course leader re appropriate subjects.
	Make up a study timetable.

Next, students are encouraged to identify likely obstacles (item 4.3) to the plan and how they might overcome these (item 4.4). The awareness of potential obstacles provides students with the opportunity to consider ways to either remove, avoid or get around obstacles should they arise (see item 4.4).

4.3	Now review your plans. What do you think are the obstacles to these plans working out for you?
A.	Getting someone to look after my child while I go to the library.
	Guilt.
	Family/commitments.
	Staff shortages at work.
	Lack of self-discipline.
	Time is restricted as I work full time and have commitments.
	Line manager is not keen to authorise study time. I feel guilty that I am passing some family/household commitments to my husband to deal with.
	Allowing myself to make excuses for not studying.
	Other pressures on time, full-time working, young family.
	Husband is understanding but need to spend time with him.

4.4	Having identified some potential obstacles, how can you remove/get around these obstacles?
A.	Fix times and stick to them.
	Speak to staff rep re study time or further up past line manager to establish a case for study time.
	Perhaps by telling someone what my intentions are.
	Set aside time and start.
	Study for frequent short periods during the week.

Students are then encouraged, in items 5.1 and 5.2, to decide when would be good times to review the implementation of the plan and what they might expect the benefits to be. In item 5.3, some students opted to review within a short period of time (for example, within a couple of days), whereas others opted for a longer review period (for example, several weeks). The decision when to review would depend on the nature and extent of each action or goal. A goal of making a study timetable (the last plan given in item 4.2.1 above) might be appropriately reviewed within a few days. Taking action to obtain study time from an employer (solution 8 in item 4.1) or negotiating at work with a line manager or higher (item 4.3) may take several weeks. In line with the theory outlined in Section 3 of the main text (see pages 12–13), control of the decision-making process continues to remain with the student.

5.1	When would be a good time to review this plan . . . within a few hours, days, weeks or months?
A.	I will review this plan . . .
	This weekend.
	In the next week.
	In two or three weeks.
	Weekly to keep me motivated.
	In two months.

Evaluate and monitor (Stage 6 of decision-making)

Armed with the reflections from items 4.3 to 5.1 in the previous stage, students completing the SAMI are next drawn to consider actions they might take if they find that one or more of their prioritised solutions have been achieved (item 5.2). Alternatively, if insufficient progress has been made at a time of evaluation, they are asked in item 5.3 how they might alter their plans in order to achieve greater progress. This is phrased to elicit a self-motivational statement such as 'I will review my goals, make them more realistic and try again'. An actual response to item 5.3 was 'Review and try to see where I am going wrong and how I can change it'. In the spirit of equipoise in motivational interviewing, another student responded 'Re-assess my reason for being on the course', demonstrating that decision-making responsibility continues to lie with the student.

5.2	If you have successfully completed the plan when you review it, consider and try to list the benefits and achievements you anticipate (you may like to give yourself a reward).
A.	Better grades.
	Peace of mind. Fulfillment.
	Just a feeling that I was managing the module – rather than it managing me.
	Obtain a degree – in turn opens doors for professional development.
	A degree!!!

5.3	If you have not been able to complete all or any of your plan when you review it, can you consider and list ways of altering or amending this in order that you are more guaranteed some progress?
A.	If I do not complete my plan I will . . .
	Review and try to see where I am going wrong and how I can change it.
	Try harder.
	Set realistic goals.
	Re-assess my reason for being on the course.
	Have to reconsider plan and assess whether current studies are important.

Theory underpinning the SAMI was discussed in Section 3 of the main text (see page 9); in the current section the design and layout of the instrument was discussed and sample student responses were given. Section 5, as follows, contains some suggested applications of the SAMI.

5. WAYS TO USE THE INSTRUMENT

An initial evaluation of the SAMI was conducted in a controlled experiment undertaken for a PhD (Duffy, 2005). This is discussed next and, from that experience, suggestions are made on how the instrument might be used in other academic settings. The point of the controlled experiment was to assess the influence of the motivational instrument (SAMI) on approaches to study and its impact on academic attainment.

Figure 1 demonstrates the experiment. Students were assigned to one of two groups, which were geographically dispersed (in that they studied on different campuses) and so had no contact with each other. Each group consisted of students in levels 1, 2 and 3 of UK degrees. As shown in the figure, students were asked in the first week of semester if they would participate in the study. At that time, it was explained that being involved meant completing a questionnaire in the next tutorial and completing a further brief questionnaire in week 11. They were advised that the week 2 activity might help with their approaches to study. They were advised also that participation was on an 'opt-in' basis and not compulsory.

Students in the control group completed the condensed ASSIST and the 'How well' question. This took less than five minutes in general. Students in the intervention group were provided in addition with a paper document that included all of the SAMI sections (Appendix 1 on page 51). On average students in the intervention group took approximately half an hour to complete this. Equal numbers of students (164) in each group returned completed, useable questionnaires in week 2.

The SAMI booklets were then taken away for photocopying and returned in week 3. This allowed students in the intervention group and the researcher to retain copies. Students were encouraged to refer to the booklet from time to time during the module as a reminder of their reflections on approach to study and decisions made. Also, copies were retained to ensure that students' completed SAMIs would be available in week 11, when they were asked to review progress. Week 11 was chosen as the students included in the study were all assessed by coursework that had to be submitted by week 12.

At this time, the intervention group re-did the condensed ASSIST. They were further asked to identify the extent to which they had achieved the goals they set in week 2 (Appendix 2 on page 69). To ensure they had this information to hand, photocopies of relevant pages of completed SAMIs were provided. Both groups of students were asked to rate their perceptions of the influence of the activity in week 2 on their approaches to study. To date, only partial analysis has been undertaken of this question. It appears that students in the intervention group were more positive about the activity. It appears that students who compete the SAMI found the activity influential. For example:

I have tried to be as honest as possible. It has helped me to review my commitment to the course.

Teaching week	Control Group	Intervention Group
Week 1	Invitation to participate	Invitation to participate
Week 2	How well? Condensed ASSIST	How well and Potential? Condensed ASSIST Motivational interview and Decision-making
Week 3		Return of completed instrument
Week 4		⋮
Week 5		⋮
Week 6		⋮
Week 7		⋮
Week 8		⋮
Week 9		⋮
Week 10		⋮
Week 11	Condensed ASSIST Evaluation of week 2 activity	Condensed ASSIST Review of achievement Evaluation of week 2 activity
Week 12		⋮
Week 13		⋮

Figure 1 The controlled experiment using the SAMI

Problems I have with this course include lack of IT skills, along with family commitments and work commitments. I would get better results if I was a full-time student or had no family or worked part time. I looked at the priorities such as not doing the housework, which was not possible, giving the family less time and support (again, not possible) or not fulfilling my work commitments (again, not possible) so I will just have to struggle on.

My biggest problem is time management and trying to cope with running a house, working and looking after kids, husband and dog! However I hope by writing down and thinking about my approach to study I have learned a few things.

It [the SAMI], made me address the issue of 'study approach' that I didn't want to tackle. Anyway, the reward bit seems to be working already, as I am off to make some tablet [a Scottish sweet commonly made in the home]. I hope I deserve it.

I didn't like doing it [the SAMI], – it made me face up to a few facts about my studying I have chosen to ignore!

Lecturers and personal tutors could apply the SAMI as was done for the intervention group, with or without the evaluative component. This is taken up next.

6. WAYS TO USE A BRIEF, SELF-ADMINISTERED INSTRUMENT

Recall that distributing and providing advice on how to complete the SAMI took only a few minutes; while completion of the instrument by students took about half an hour. Thus the experience gained in the controlled experiment suggests that self-administered instruments can be designed that require little time to implement. Further, the analysis of the data gathered in the controlled experiment supports the hypothesis that involvement in the intervention-group activities in weeks 1, 2 and 3 influences approaches to study and academic outcomes (Duffy, 2005; Duffy and Rimmer, 2005). Thus, for relatively minor erosions of class time, changes of study behaviour occurred.

Further, between the second and eleventh weeks of semester, the only intervention received was to have completed SAMIs returned in week 3. It was made clear that students should look back from time to time at their SAMI responses. Consequently, it is feasible to suggest that students might undertake the SAMI intervention with little or no staff involvement. In the latter case, students would be completely reliant on themselves to ensure that each stage of the instrument is completed fully.

If some staff involvement is thought appropriate following the administration of the SAMI, this might not need to be extensive or even to involve class time. Rather, it could consist of gentle reminders at one or two tutorials to look back at the completed instrument and monitor progress with action plans. Alternatively, this could be prompted when students log on to a virtual learning environment associated with their course, or e-mails could be sent to a class to suggest student-centred review of completed SAMIs.

In some cases, greater levels of staff input might be beneficial in aiding reflection on students' responses. For example, having completed the instrument, a personal tutor, lecturer or academic adviser could arrange to discuss the student's responses in a one-to-one follow-up interview. This may serve to highlight key areas of concern and assist the student in focussing on action plans and evaluating progress towards intended outcomes. In this form of additional support, staff should adopt an interview approach that is consistent with the principles of motivational interviewing. Moreover, students may be more inclined to work to meet the goals that they set if they know there will be a meeting with a staff member to evaluate progress.

Another possibility, which directly parallels the experiences of the intervention group, is that the SAMI is administered in small classes, such as tutorials. One specific area where this may be beneficial is that tutors might ask students to concentrate especially on generating multiple alternative solutions. In the controlled experiment, most students generated no more than four alternatives. Tutor emphasis on this aspect might encourage putting more time into this part of the SAMI, hopefully leading to better quality solutions (see Section 4 of the main text, page 33). In subsequent classes, students might be prompted to undertake a few minutes' review of progress, regardless of when the students recorded that they would evaluate. If a review is not appropriate at the time but a tutor suggests one might be considered, the students would retain the authority to disregard the call. Alternatively, tutors might simply remind students that they set review dates, perhaps along with reminding students of looming submission or examination dates to refresh ambivalence.

It is likely that lecturers and teachers will think of variations of SAMI administration that are appropriate to their environments and which have not been mentioned here. Moreover, it is likely also that lecturers and teachers can devise variations of the SAMI content that improve the relevance of an intervention for their students. In part, it underpins the invitation to become involved in the ongoing development and research on self-administered, brief interventions aimed at improving study habits. In addition to adding to the evidence base, lecturers and teachers contributing to the evolution of SAMI-like instruments might use the SAMI as a means to understand better the conflicting demands that many modern students confront (see Section 2 of the main text, pages 4–6).

7. CONCLUSION

The aim in this work has been to make available and promote the use of motivational interviewing in forms that students might self-administer. As set out in Section 3 of the main text, the construction of the SAMI (Self Administered Motivational Instrument) was guided by findings on learning styles, motivational interviewing, brief interventions and decision-making. In a controlled experiment (Duffy, 2005; Duffy and Rimmer, 2005) it was found that doing the SAMI was associated with changes in approaches to study; in particular a small to medium effect size was found for students who completed the SAMI (Cohen, 1969); and greater strategic scores on a condensed version of the ASSIST instrument (Entwistle *et al.*, 2000) were associated with a greater likelihood of attaining one of the top grades of A or B1. As the application of the SAMI in a controlled experiment was low cost (in terms of class time and staff resources, see Section 4, page 21), the small to medium effect and the positive influence on grades might be considered to be a reasonable return.

The broad conclusion is that a SAMI can elicit positive changes in approaches to study that impact directly on study outcomes. However, we would not wish to suggest that the form of the instrument, or indeed the components of the instrument, cannot be improved. There are many possible ways in which the SAMI might be modified in the search for a more effective instrument. We have already had suggestions that the use of a learning-style inventory is inappropriate, because the link between scores on an inventory and academic outcomes are not always substantiated; and reinforcing ambivalence induced in an earlier section of the instrument might be more effective using some other means of raising awareness.

Another area for investigation is to research the best means of stimulating student engagement with a SAMI. In the previous section a number of suggestions was made, ranging from students using it independently of any external intervention, to teacher involvement on a one-to-one basis or one-to-class basis. A third suggestion is to study the effects of a SAMI on students' likelihood of progression and retention.

Another research suggestion is to investigate environmental and background factors that might mediate the effectiveness of a SAMI. A student's concerns about study is likely to differ depending on their background, ability and the environment in which study occurs. Further, the point about a self-administered motivational instrument is that students have the opportunity to improve their approaches in a manner and pace appropriate to them, independent of advice or leadership from an external source. Given this, is it likely therefore that a SAMI-like instrument might be more effective for some students than for others?

Our intention in writing this resource was to make the instrument available. Indeed, we hope that the use of it by your students will provide insight into the use and modification of the SAMI format. To this end we would be delighted to hear of your experiences in applying the SAMI and in collaborating with you in its evolution. We can be contacted via:

Dr Tim Duffy
Director of Distance Learning
School of Health, Nursing and Midwifery
University of the West of Scotland
Paisley Campus
Paisley
PA12BE
Tel 0141 848 3952
Tim.Duffy@uws.ac.uk

References

Adair, J. (1985) *Effective Decision Making.* Reading: Cox and Wyman

Adair, J. (1997) *Decision making and problem solving, Training Extras.* London: Institute of Personnel and Development

Allinson, C. and Hayes, J. (1996) 'The Cognitive Style Index'. *Journal of Management Studies*, 33: 119–135

Apter, M., Mallows, R. and Williams, S. (1998) 'The development of the Motivational Style Profile'. *Personality and Individual Differences*, 24(1): 7–18

Astin, A. (1984) 'Student involvement: A developmental theory for higher education'. *Journal of College Student Development*, 25: 297–308

Astin, A. (1998) 'The changing American college student; thirty year trends, 1966–1996'. *The Review of Higher Education*, 21(2): 151–165

Baty, P. (2005) 'QAA tells Leeds Met to close loophole', *Times Higher Education Supplement* 1690, 06 May

Bean, J. and Metzner, B. (1985) 'A conceptual model of non-traditional undergraduate student attrition'. *Review of Educational Research*, 55: 485–540

Bien, T.H., Miller, W.R. and Tonigan, J.S. (1993) 'Brief interventions for alcohol problems: a review'. *Addiction*, 88(3): 315–335

Biggs, J.B. (1988) 'The role of metacognition in enhancing learning'. *Australian Journal of Education*, 32: 127–138

Biggs, J.B. (1993) 'What do inventories of students' learning processes really measure? A theoretical review and clarification'. *Educational Psychology*, 63: 3–9

Bourgeois, E., Duke, C., Guyot, J.-L. and Merrill, B. (1999) *The Adult University.* Buckingham: Society for Research into Higher Education

Brennan, J., Callendar, C., Duaso, A., Little, B. and Van Dyke, R. (2005) 'Survey of higher education students' attitudes to debt and term-time working and their impact on attainment: A report to Universities UK and HEFCE by the Centre for Higher Education Research and Information (CHERI) and London South Bank University'. London: Universities UK

Burke, B.L., Arkowitz, H. and Dunn, C. (2002) 'The efficacy of motivational interviewing and its adaptations. What we know so far'. In W.R. Miller and S. Rollnick (eds) *Motivational Interviewing: Preparing People for Change.* New York: Guildford Press

Burke, B., Arkowitz, H. and Menchola, M. (2001) 'The efficacy of motivational interviewing: A meta-analysis of controlled clinical trials'. *Journal of Consulting and Clinical Psychology*, 71: 843–861

Byrnes, J.P. (2001) *Cognitive Development and Learning in Instructional Contexts*. New Jersey: Allyn and Bacon

Callendar, C. (2005) 'Too much like hard work', The *Guardian*, November 29. Available at **http://education.guardian.co.uk/higher/comment/story/0,9828, 1652794,00.html** (Accessed: 25 January 2008)

Chang, R.Y. and Kelly, P.K. (1993) *Step-by-step Problem Solving*. California: Richard Chang Associates.

Cloonan, M. (2004) 'Notions of flexibility in UK higher education: core and periphery re-visited'. *Higher Education Quarterly*, 58: 176–197

Coffield, F., Moseley, D., Hall, E. and Ecclesstone, K. (2004) *Learning Styles and Pedagogy in Post-16 Learning: A Systematic and Critical Review*. London: Learning and Skills Research Council

Cohen, J. (1969) *Statistical Power Analysis for the Behavioural Sciences*. NY: Academic Press

Dansereau, D.F. (1985) 'Learning Strategy Research', in J.W. Segal, S.F. Chipman and R. Glaser (eds) *Thinking and Learning Skills. Relating Instruction to Research*, 1: 209–239. London: Lawrence Erlbaum Associates

Donnelly, M., McCormack, D. and Rimmer, R. (2007) 'Load and academic attainment in two business schools'. *Assessment and Evaluation in Higher Education*, 32(6): 613–630

Duff, A. (1997) 'A note on the reliability and validity of a 30-item version of Enwistle and Tait's revised approaches to studying inventory'. *British Journal of Educational Psychology*, 67: 529–539

Duffy, T. (2005) 'Improving approaches to study using a Self Administered Motivational Instrument (SAMI)'. Paisley: University of Paisley

Duffy, T. (1994) 'Brief interventions and their role in relation to more intensive treatment of alcohol problems. Addictions Update'. Health Promotion Department, Greater Glasgow Health Board, Scotland

Duffy, T. and Rimmer, R. (2005) 'Learning style and academic attainment among nursing students', in M. Osborne, J. Gallacher and R. Edwards (eds) *What a Difference a Pedagogy Makes: Researching Lifelong Learning and Teaching*, June: 126–136, Glasgow: Centre for Research in Lifelong Learning. 1-903661-72-2

Dunn, C., Deroo, L. and Rivara, F.P. (2001) 'The use of brief interventions adapted from motivational interviewing across behavioural domains: a systematic review'. *Addiction*, 96: 1725–1742

D'Zurrilla, T. and Goldfried, M. (1971) 'Problem solving and behavior modification'. *Journal of Abnormal Psychology*, 78: 107–126

Entwistle, N., Tait, H. and McCune, V. (2000) 'Patterns of response to an approaches to studying inventory across contrasting groups and contexts'. *European Journal of the Psychology of Education*, 15: 33–48

Gibbs, G. (1997) *Improving Student Learning: Theory and Practice*. Oxford: The Oxford Centre for Staff Development

Harlen, W. and Crick, R.D. (2003) 'Testing and Motivating for Learning'. *Assessment in Education*, 10(2): 169–207

Heather, N. (2005) 'Motivational interviewing: Is it all our clients need?' *Addiction Research and Theory*, 13(1): 1–18

Herrmann, N. (1996) *The Whole Brain Business Book*. New York: McGraw-Hill

Houston, M. and Rimmer, R. (2005) 'A comparison of academic outcomes for business and other students'. *International Journal of Management Education*, 4(3): 11–19

Houston, M. and Rimmer, R. (2007) 'Transition from first to second semester: trading off study, work and life', in *The times they are a-changin': researching transitions in lifelong learning, Proceedings of the CRLL Conference*. Stirling: Center for Research in Lifelong Learning

Houston, M. and Rimmer, R. (2008) 'School mathematics and university outcomes'. To appear in M. Grove and C. Marr (eds) *Addressing the Quantitative Skills Gap: Establishing and Sustaining Cross-curricular Mathematical Support in Higher Education*. Glasgow: HEA Mathematics, Statistics and Operations Research

Houston, M., Knox, H. and Rimmer, R. (2007) 'Wider access and progression among full-time students'. *Higher Education*, 53(1): 107–146

Kuh, G. (1998) 'How are we doing? Tracking the quality of the undergraduate experience from the 1960s to the present'. *Review of Higher Education*, 22(2): 90–120

Kuh, G. (2001) 'Assessing what really matters of student learning'. *Change*, May/June

Leppel, K. (2001) 'The impact of major on college persistence among freshmen'. *Higher Education*, 41(3): 327–342

Lowe, J. and Gayle, V. (2007) 'Exploring the work/life/study balance: the experience of higher education students in a Scottish further education college'. *Journal of Further and Higher Education*, 31(3): 225–238

LSDA (2003) *Learner Motivation and Barriers to Participation in Post-16 Learning. A Brief Review of the Literature*. London: Learning and Skills Development Agency

LSRC, (2004) *Do Summative Assessment and Testing have a Positive or Negative Effect on Post-16 Learners' Motivation for Learning in the Learning and Skills Sector? A Review of the Literature on Assessment in Post-compulsory Education in the UK*. London: Learning and Skills Research Centre

LSRC (2004) *Learning Styles for Post-16 Learners. What do we Know?* London: Learning and Skills Research Centre

March, J.G. (ed.) (1999) *The Pursuit of Organizational Intelligence*. New York: Blackwell

Martin, E. and Ramsden, P. (1987) 'Learning skills or skill in learning?' In J.T.E. Richardson, M.W. Eysenck and D.W. Piper (eds) *Student Learning, Research in Education and Cognitive Psychology*. Milton Keynes: The Society for Research into Higher Education and Open University Press

Marzano, R.J. (1998) *A Theory-based Meta-analysis of Research on Instruction*. Aurora, CO: Mid-continent Regional Educational Laboratory

McInnes, C. (2001) 'Signs of disengagement? The changing undergraduate experience in Australian universities', Inaugural professorial lecture, University of Melbourne, Australia: Centre for the Study of Higher Education, Faculty of Education

Merrill, B. (2001) 'Learning and Teaching in Universities: perspectives from adult learners and lecturers'. *Teaching in Higher Education*, 6:(1): 5–17

Miller, W.R. and Rollnick, S. (2002) *Motivational Interviewing. Preparing People for Change*. New York: Guildford Press

Morgan-Klein, B. (2003) 'Negotiating the climbing frame: flexibility and access in Scottish higher education'. *European Journal of Education*, 38(1): 41–54

Morgan-Klein, B. and Gray, P. (2000) 'Flexible trends: researching part-time students and flexibility in higher education'. *Scottish Journal of Adult and Continuing Education*, 6(10): 41–57

Morris, H. (2000) 'The origins, forms and effects of modularization and semesterisation in ten UK-based business schools'. *Higher Education Quarterly*, 54(3): 239–258

Murphy, M., Morgan-Klein, B., Osborne, M. and Gallacher, J. (2003) *Widening Access to Higher Education*. Glasgow and Stirling: Centre for Research in Lifelong Learning

Myers, I.B. and McCaulley M.H. (1998) *Manual: A Guide to the Development and Use of the Myers-Briggs Type Indicator*. Palo Alto, CA: Consulting Psychologists Press

Newman, M. (2008) 'Fees do not buy a guaranteed degree'. *Times Higher Education*, 10 January, 14

Nonis, S., Philhours, M. and Huddson, I. (2006) 'Where does the time go? A diary approach to business and marketing students' time use'. *Journal of Marketing Education*, 28: 121–134

Noonan, W.C. and Moyers, T.B. (1997) 'Motivational interviewing: A review'. *Journal of Substance Misuse*, 2: 8–16

Patrick, W. (2001) 'Estimating first-year attrition rates: an application of multilevel modelling using categorical variables'. *Research in Higher Education* 27: 15–38

Pfeffer, J. and Fong, C. (2004) 'The business school "business": some lessons from the US experience'. *Journal of Management Studies*, 41(8): 1501–1520

Quality Assurance Agency (QAA) (2004) Leeds Metropolitan University: Institutional Audit, **http://www.qaa.ac.uk/reviews/reports/institutional/leedsmet05/ RG111LeedsMet Uni.pdf** (Accessed: 1 December 2007)

Ramsden, P., Beswick, D. and Bowden, J. (1986) 'Effects of learning skills interventions on first year university students' learning'. *Human Learning*, 5: 151–164

Ramsden, P., Beswick, D. and Bowden, J. (1987) 'Learning processes and learning skills' in J.T.E. Richardson, M.W. Eysenck and D.W. Piper (eds) *Student Learning. Research in Education and Cognitive Psychology*. Milton Keynes: The Society for Research into Higher Education and Open University Press

Reeves, A. and Rimmer, R. (2008) 'Explaining performance in an Executive MBA', to appear in *International Journal of Management Education*

Richardson, J. and Woodley, A. (2003) 'Another look at the role of age, gender and subject as predictors of academic attainment in higher education'. *Studies in Higher Education*, 28(4): 475–490

Rimmer, R. and Rimmer, S. (1997) 'Employment breaks, pay and career development among Australian women'. *Gender, Work and Organisation*, 4: 202–217

Rollnick, S. and Miller, W.R. (1995) 'What is MI?'. *Behavioural and Cognitive Psychotherapy*, 23: 325–334

Schuller, T. and Bamford, C. (2000) 'A social capital approach to the analysis of continuing education: evidence from the UK learning society research project'. *Oxford Review of Education*, 26(1): 6–19

SQW (2006) 'Demand for flexible and innovative types of higher education'. Report to HEFCE by SQW Ltd and Taylor Nelson Sofres. Cambridge: SQW

Tait, H. and Entwistle, N.J. (1996) 'Identifying students at risk through ineffective study strategies'. *Higher Education*, 31(1): 97–116

Tinto, V. (1975) 'Dropout from higher education: a theoretical synthesis of recent research'. *Review of Educational Research*, 45(1): 89–125

Velleman, R. (1991) 'Alcohol and drug problems' in W. Dryden and R. Rentoul (eds) *Clinical Problems: a Cognitive-Behavioural Approach*. London: Routledge

Vermunt, J.D. (1996) 'Metacognitive, cognitive and affective aspects of learning styles and strategies: a phenomenographic analysis'. *Higher Education*, 31: 25–50

Whetten, D. and Cameron, K. (2002) *Developing Management Skills*. Upper Saddle River: Prentice Hall

Weick, K. (1984) 'Small wins'. *American Psychologist*, 39: 40–49.

Woodley, A., Thompson, M. and Cowan, J. (1992), *Factors Affecting Non-completion Rates in Scottish Universities*. Milton Keynes: Institute of Educational Technology, Open University

Yorke, M. (2002) 'Degree classification in English, Welsh and Northern Irish universities: trends 1994–5 to 1998–99'. *Higher Education Quarterly*, 56(1): 92–108

Appendix 1: The Self Administered Motivational Instrument (SAMI)

Student Name . . . .

Matriculation number . . . .

Produced by _____

This booklet has been prepared to help you in any decisions you may make about your studying. After you have filled it in, you may find it useful to refer to it from time to time. The first thing to consider is how well you think you are doing with your study at the moment.

SECTION 1

1.1

On a score from 1-9, how well do think you are doing with your study (where 1 is 'not very well' and 9 is 'very well')? Place an X in the box below the appropriate number.

Not very well   Very well

1	2	3	4	5	6	7	8	9

On a score from 1-9, how well do think you could score if you really tried your best (where 1 is 'not very well' and 9 is 'very well')? Place an X in the box below the appropriate number.

Not very well   Very well

1	2	3	4	5	6	7	8	9

Now have a look at the above scores and compare them.

1.2	If the above scores differ, in what way does this bother you (if at all)?
A.	

SECTION 2

This next section asks you to indicate your relative agreement or disagreement with comments about studying that have been made by other students. You are asked to work through these items quickly, giving your immediate reaction to each one.

2.1

In the highlighted shaded column on the right below, rate each question either 1, 2, 3, 4 or 5 using the following criteria.

Agree	5
Agree somewhat	4
Unsure	3
Somewhat disagree	2
Disagree	1

I'm not prepared just to accept things I'm told: I have to think them out for myself.	
One way or another I manage to get hold of books or whatever I need for studying.	
Sometimes I find myself thinking about ideas from the course when I'm doing other things.	
I make sure I find conditions for studying which let me get on with my work easily.	
I try to relate ideas I come across to other topics or other courses whenever possible.	
I put a lot of effort into making sure I have the most important details at my fingertips.	
I organise my study time carefully to make the best use of it.	
When I'm reading an article or book, I try to work out for myself exactly what's being said.	
I know what I want to get out of this course and I'm determined to achieve it.	
I usually set out to understand for myself the meaning of what we have to learn.	
I work hard when I'm studying and generally manage to keep my mind on what I'm doing.	

When I'm working on a new topic, I try to see in my own mind how all the ideas fit together.	
It's important to me to feel I'm doing as well as I really can on the course here.	
Ideas in course books or articles often set me off on long chains of thought about what I'm reading.	
I think I'm quite systematic and organised in the way I go about studying.	
When I'm reading I examine the details carefully to see how they fit in with what's being said.	
I generally try to make good use of my time during the day.	
It's important to me to be able to follow the argument or see the reasoning behind something.	
I work steadily throughout the course, rather than leaving everything until the last minute.	
I look at the evidence carefully and then try to reach my own conclusion about things I'm studying.	
Total	

Now calculate your total by adding the numbers in the shaded area on the right hand column above. Review your total score for the above questions. The minimum score you can obtain is 20, the maximum is 100. There are research indications that there is a link between a student's score and the marks they are likely to be awarded in their coursework assignments. Those scoring highly would generally perform well in assessed work, while those scoring low would perform less well.

2.2	What do you like/dislike about your total score for the above questions?

A.

SECTION 3

Now let's have a look at some issues relating to your own approach to study.

3.1	The problems I have with my approach to studying are:

A.

3.2	What is it that worries you about these difficulties?
A.	

Now let's have a look at some beneficial aspects of your current approach to study.

3.3	If I continue to study in the way I do now, the benefits would be:
A.	

3.4	In what way are these aspects beneficial to you?

A.

Let us now have a look at some of the drawbacks to your current approach to study.

3.5	If I continue to study in the way I do now, the drawbacks would be:

A.

3.6   What is it that particularly concerns you about these drawbacks?

A.

3.7   If I changed my approach to studying the drawbacks would be:

A.

3.8	What is it that particularly concerns you about these drawbacks?
A.	

3.9	If I changed my approach to studying the benefits would be:
A.	

If you decide to change your approach to studying there may be some obstacles or difficulties in making this change. Now consider some of these obstacles.

3.10	What are the main obstacles to me changing my approach to studying?
A.	

There are likely to be a range of pros and cons when considering a change to your approach to studying. Having reviewed some of these, now identify the main reasons for you making a change.

3.11	The reasons I have for changing my approach to study are:
A.	

Having considered a range of issues in relation to your approach to study, now try to focus on the key problem you face in this area.

3.12	So what really is the main problem in relation to your approach to study? Be very, very specific.

A.

SECTION 4

4.1

Now have another look at your answer to question 3.12.
Stand back and try to be objective.
Try to list as many possible ways of resolving this problem (around 10 ideas).

Solutions	Please write in this column what you think may be a possible solution to what you have identified as your main problem. Ignore the two columns on the right for a minute, you will be asked to consider these shortly.	Delete	Prioritise
Solution 1			

Solution 2		
Solution 3		
Solution 4		
Solution 5		
Solution 6		
Solution 7		
Solution 8		
Solution 9		
Solution 10		

Now read again the main problem you are trying to resolve. Bearing this in mind, get rid of the poor options.

> Place an 'x' in the 'Delete' column above to identify solutions you want to get rid of.

Have another look at your list. This time try to prioritise those solutions you have not deleted.

> In the 'Prioritise' column above:
>
> Mark with a 1 the solution you think is most appropriate/relevant.
> Mark with a 2 the solution you think is the next most appropriate/relevant.
> Mark with a 3 the next most appropriate/relevant.

4.2

Now take the number 1 solution.

4.2.1	How can you put this solution into action in a realistic and achievable manner? Develop a plan by completing the following sentence:
A.	I will put this into action by . . .

Now take the number 2 solution.

4.2.2	How can you put this solution into action in a realistic and achievable manner? Develop a plan by completing the following sentence:
A.	I will put this into action by . . .

Now take the number 3 solution.

4.2.3	How can you put this solution into action in a realistic and achievable manner? Develop a plan by completing the following sentence:
A.	I will put this into action by . . .

4.3	Now review your plans. What do you think are the obstacles to these plans working out for you?
A.	

4.4	Having identified some potential obstacles how can you remove/get around these obstacles?
A.	

You should now have a clear idea of what you wish to do in order to change your approach to study.

SECTION 5

Now take a minute to identify when you should review progress on your plan.

5.1	When would be a good time to review this plan . . . within a few hours, days, weeks or months?
A.	I will review this plan . . .

5.2	If you have successfully completed the plan when you review it, consider and try to list the benefits and achievements you anticipate (you may like to give yourself a reward):
A.	

5.3	If you have not been able to complete all or any of your plan when you review it, can you consider and list ways of altering, amending this in order that you are more guaranteed some progress?
A.	

Thank you and good luck with your studies.

Appendix 2: Revisiting the SAMI

Student Name . . . .

Matriculation Number . . . .

> In the highlighted shaded column on the right below, rate each question either 1, 2, 3, 4 or 5 using the following criteria.
>
> | | |
> |---|---|
> | Agree | 5 |
> | Agree somewhat | 4 |
> | Unsure | 3 |
> | Somewhat disagree | 2 |
> | Disagree | 1 |

I'm not prepared just to accept things I'm told: I have to think them out for myself.	
One way or another I manage to get hold of books or whatever I need for studying.	
Sometimes I find myself thinking about ideas from the course when I'm doing other things.	
I make sure I find conditions for studying which let me get on with my work easily.	
I try to relate ideas I come across to other topics or other courses whenever possible.	
I put a lot of effort into making sure I have the most important details at my fingertips.	
I organise my study time carefully to make the best use of it.	
When I'm reading an article or book, I try to work out for myself exactly what's being said.	
I know what I want to get out of this course and I'm determined to achieve it.	

The SAMI may be photocopied for use by the purchaser within their own institution only, under the terms of the institution's photocopying licence. (Tait and Entwistle, 1996; Entwistle *et al.*, 2000)

I usually set out to understand for myself the meaning of what we have to learn.	
I work hard when I'm studying and generally manage to keep my mind on what I'm doing.	
When I'm working on a new topic, I try to see in my own mind how all the ideas fit together.	
It's important to me to feel I'm doing as well as I really can on the course here.	
Ideas in course books or articles often set me off on long chains of thought about what I'm reading.	
I think I'm quite systematic and organised in the way I go about studying.	
When I'm reading I examine the details carefully to see how they fit in with what's being said.	
I generally try to make good use of my time during the day.	
It's important to me to be able to follow the argument or see the reasoning behind something.	
I work steadily throughout the course, rather than leaving everything until the last minute.	
I look at the evidence carefully and then try to reach my own conclusion about things I'm studying.	
Total	

When you completed an earlier interview schedule, you identified some areas in which you aimed to improve your approach to study.

Please see the document you completed earlier.
For the three action plans you identified, please indicate the degree of progress you have made in carrying out your plan (see 4.2.1, 4.2.2 and 4.2.3)

Solution number 1.

Please place an X in the box below the appropriate number you believe identifies the degree of success you have had in achieving your planned action.

Not at all   Completely

1	2	3	4	5	6	7	8	9

Solution number 2.

Please place an X in the box below the appropriate number you believe identifies the degree of success you have had in achieving your planned action.

Not at all   Completely

1	2	3	4	5	6	7	8	9

Solution number 3.

Please place an X in the box below the appropriate number you believe identifies the degree of success you have had in achieving your planned action.

Not at all   Completely

1	2	3	4	5	6	7	8	9

And finally:

How influential has your completion of the SAMI been in enabling you to improve your approach to your study? Please place an X in the box below the appropriate number

Not influential   Highly influential

1	2	3	4	5	6	7	8	9	10

Thank you and good luck with your studies.